"DON'T GIVE UP, YOU HAVE FOUND US" © 2012

by

Gary Heesch

Twenty years of Research and Clinical Trials with thousands of patients all over the world with a 90% success rate in eradicating most skin disorders from Psoriasis, Molluscum, Cystic Acne, and many others with no side effects of any consequence.

Released by Medisys Research Group, Inc.
1575 Valley View Circle
Springville, UT 84663
Phone: 801-491-0177

A Utah Corporation

Patents Awarded in 2001

Restrictions: Information in this book is owned by Medisys Research Group, Inc. – a Utah Corporation - and its use is intended for those who purchase this book *"Don't Give Up, You Have Found Us."*

No information in this book may be reprinted, published, or sold without the express written permission of Medisys Research Group, Inc. of Utah.

Any organization, entity, and/or person doing so will be held liable under existing State, United States, and International Copyright and Patent laws and statutes.

Exception

Any medical practitioner licensed to give his/her patients prescriptions for medications is free to reprint or modify any of the treatment protocols for a specific patient with a skin disorder as contained in this book.

Disclaimer

Because Medisys Research Group has no direct control over a physician or the patient's use of the therapeutic protocols suggested in this booklet, we cannot be responsible or guarantee the patient's success with their skin disorder.

CONTENTS

Pages

ANTIDOTAL STORY	1
INTRODUCTION	3
CLINICAL AND PHYSICIAN TRIALS	3
JOURNEY INTO HELL	4
FIRST MEDICAL CLINIC	7
THEORETICAL PREMISE	9
COMMENTS	13
PROTOCOLS FOR SKIN DISORDERS	13-28
REFERENCES : CLINICAL TRIALS AND CERTIFICATIONS	
Psoriasis	13
Molluscum	15
Cystic Acne / Acne	16
Rosacea	18
Folliculitis	19
Athlete's Foot	20
Cold Sores / Canker Sores	21
Eczema	23
Unexplained Skin Diseases	24
Seborrhea	24
Wound Healing	26
Skin Rejuvenation	27

DON'T GIVE UP, YOU HAVE FOUND US © 2012

Still a Mystery

As the CEO, and involved in the research to find cures for a broad range of skin disorders, I very seldom visited our clinic in Midvale, Utah. But in the spring of 2000, I did.

As I walked in, one of the medical assistants pulled me aside, and in a pleading, but firm voice said, "Gary, please come and see the patient in one of the patient rooms." I said, "What is the problem?" She said, "Please don't ask; just come with me."

As we walked into the room, I had no idea what to expect. In the patient's chair sat a well-built, handsome, Polynesian man about fifty years of age. In three chairs along the wall sat two teenage boys and a beautiful teenage girl. Everything seemed normal, nothing unusual, until I introduced myself and asked, "What is the problem here?"

The medical assistant looked at me in stark disbelief, and the father of these three young people would not look at me.

No one was saying a word, and then I saw. I tried my best to maintain my composure as I looked in disbelief at the patient's right cheek, and on down to his neck. It looked as though someone had applied white cake frosting smoothly over these areas of his skin.

In my sixteen years of research I had never seen anything so unusual, and it was somewhat uncomfortable for me, as I had no idea what could possibly have caused such a condition.

The feeling of despair was so strong in the room; all I could do was try my best to be professional; and so I asked the patient if he would introduce himself and his children. The silence was broken, but the strong feeling of despair was ever there in the face of the father and his children.

It was time to start asking questions. Little did I know what was coming. "Sir," I asked, "Have you seen any physicians about your problem?" He answered, "Yes, he had seen two doctors, and the second one said there was nothing that could be done to help him, and worst of all, the skin disorder would continue to spread."

The patient then said, "In my culture, our appearance is very important to us, and I would rather not live than have this for the rest of my life." I got the message loud and clear. I looked at his children; their eyes as big as saucers, leaning forward in their chairs as they understood exactly what he was saying.

My first thought was that I'd have to lighten the mood in the room if anything at all was going to be accomplished. This patient was a big man, and I was not sure what I could get away with. Where I got the courage is another story, but I asked him how much money he had in the bank. In a low, firm, don't play with me voice he said, "What business is that of yours?" I stood firm with my bluff and said, "It's my business because I'm going to charge you one million dollars to get rid of this problem you have." It worked! I saw his eyes light up, and a big smile made all the despair evaporate from the room.

Copyright 1996 Medisys Research Group, Inc.

He knew I was joking and said, "Do you really think you can help me?" I lied through my teeth, but I had to continue the bluff if for no other reason than to stall for time, because this patient was planning to take his life way before he ever came to our clinic. We were his last stop – no more tries after us.

Once things calmed down, it was time to get a history on this patient to see if anything at all would give me a clue to his condition. The more questions I asked him, the less I knew. I was in a corner all by myself, and there was no way out but to try everything I had learned in sixteen years.

When inspiration comes, you know it. In that room, in just a few minutes I wrote down a therapy protocol. I went over it with the patient and the medical assistant who knew how high the stakes were, and the dye was cast.

What this man had is still a mystery, but in approximately eight weeks I received a telephone call from the clinic. Our patient who lived three hundred miles away in St. George, Utah had come in for his last visit, and was completely cured – a word we do not use lightly in medicine. I was told that he would like to see me on my next visit to St. George.

I had an occasion to visit St. George, and we went to lunch. He then revealed his position as one of the founders of a well-known Utah company, and with tears in his eyes he thanked me for saving his life. He has no idea how relieved I was from the whole experience; and how happy I was for him and his three beautiful children.

Copyright 1996 Medisys Research Group, Inc.

Introduction

An introduction I guess should be just that – an introduction to the things you're going to learn; not just about the therapeutic protocols that will successfully treat the more common disorders, such as psoriasis, molluscum, cystic acne, eczema, etc., but even the most ugly, outrageous skin diseases that have no name. But also, you will learn about the work, the years of sacrifices that go into medical research when you have no idea what you're really getting into, and how it will all end, because to be honest, after twenty-five years, we are still learning, and it hasn't ended yet.

So, whether you are a person looking for a solution to your own problem, or a physician who wants to learn for the well being of your own patients; it's now in your hands. If you read this whole book, and not just the protocols, most of you will sleep at night, your anxiety will fade away, you will be able to live the normal life you never thought would be possible again. So don't cry anymore; you have found what you have been looking and praying for.

Clinical Trials

The first clinical trials were done in cooperation with a major producer of skin care products which most of you reading this have had in your home at one time or another.

These trials focused on cystic to moderate acne, and patients with eczema conditions. These trials were conducted at the Gresham Medical Center in Gresham, Oregon beginning in 1985. The age range of patients involved ranged from seven years old to fifty.

The following report by Malcolm MacGregor, M.D. at the conclusion of the trials (See References: *Clinical Trials*).

Ernst & Young Audit

Over one year after the clinical trials were completed, a request was made for Ernst & Young, out of their Chicago firm, to conduct a medical audit to confirm the results of the clinical trials. Because the audit is long and cumbersome, I have included for the satisfaction of the reader only the final letter from Ernst & Young. It should be noted that in the audit *itself*, it states that the patients experienced a "cure," and were symptom free. See References: *Clinical Trials and Certification*.

M-H Medisco Trials

In 1991, agreements were signed with M-H Medisco, a Utah Corp., to conduct studies with practicing physicians in different disciplines of medicine to determine if they could replicate the results achieved at the Gresham Medical Center in Gresham, Oregon. The second goal of this study was to determine if the physicians, unsupervised and with only the protocols, could achieve success with their patients. Their conclusions are summarized in the reference section.

Copyright 1996 Medisys Research Group, Inc.

Journey into Hell

During the Gresham Medical Center Trials, and after the Ernst & Young audit, I had some moments of inspiration that gave me the confidence to believe that other skin diseases could be challenged.

To do this kind of investigative research required money. Having been trained as an Epidemiologist by U.S. Public Health gave me some credibility, but not enough to make anyone except relatives and friends comfortable with providing much in the way of funding. Some months I had funding; other months I was broke. Our church helped us out, and my wife for the first time in twenty-five years went to work full time.

With three children and a grandchild with us, things looked pretty desperate. In spite of these circumstances, I was determined to continue my research. My wife said my problem was my ego, some said I was foolishly stubborn, and others said I had no idea what I was getting into, and they were right.

After four years of desperate ups and downs, my car was repossessed. Shortly after the car was taken, one of my younger sisters called and wanted me to go with her to look at a van at a large car dealership. We did not find what she was looking for. As we were leaving the dealership, we walked by a GMC Jimmy. I sopped to look at the interior. It was a three-year-old 1986 model and looked like new. I had never paid more than two thousand dollars for a car as I always thought new cars were a poor investment; they wanted twelve thousand for the Jimmy.

As I was looking inside at the beautiful four-wheel drive GMC, a man came up behind me and asked if I would like to take it for a ride. I laughed and said, "No, I was just admiring the car, and it was way out of my ability to buy such a vehicle." I explained to him what I did for a living, and was without funds to even keep up my research. For some reason I will never know, he said, "If you would like to have it, I will run it through and see if you qualify." I laughed again and said that my credit couldn't be any worse than it was. He said, "Never mind, I'm pretty good at what I do, and I think you're a good bet." I said, "Please don't waste your time." He said, "Just give me a little information I need, and trust me."

At that moment I thought, I need a car, but twelve thousand dollars, even if by some miracle he could pull it off, in two or three months it will just be repossessed and that could cost him his job. But then I thought, why worry; my getting approved was not even a possibility.

Two days later the phone rang and it was the fellow at the dealership. He said, "Come and pick up your GMC Jimmy." I did not know how to respond; getting the car was not even a consideration. My first thought was — get the car, at least you will have transportation for two or three months. I said I would be over in the afternoon which gave me some time to reflect on the whole thing for a while.

With all that I had accomplished so far, I was not going to give up, and if I was not going to give up, it meant that somewhere, somehow I was going to secure more funding. I picked up the GMC that afternoon; drove it home, and just parked it in the garage so no one could see I had it.

This all happened in 1989. Shortly after getting the Jimmy, my wife announced that she was filing for divorce after twenty-seven years. I tried to talk her out of it, but she was hooked on some guy where she worked. As luck would have it, I did receive some funding. I made a major decision. I packed up the Jimmy and left for Utah where I had a son living, and a few close friends. I know it sounds harsh, but if I wasn't wanted, I learned in my early years to cut out and get a change of scenery. Continuing my research could be done in Utah just as well as in Oregon.

By the way, I did not let the good fellow down at the car dealership. I paid the Jimmy off, and I will forever be grateful to him for taking such a gamble on me and possibly his job. May God bless him.

Moving to Utah meant that I had to establish new contacts, invent some way to establish a clinic to conduct more studies in my attempt to investigate a broad range of skin disorders. I didn't know how this was going to happen; I just knew I was not going to give up.

I had been in Utah about three months and was running low on money. My three children were still at home with their mother and were calling me every day and telling me that their mother was always absent from the house and she was spending the money I sent to buy herself an expensive bicycle, and there was very little food in the house.

After three months, the children were desperate and wanted to know if they could come to Utah and live with me. Growing up, they always lived in a comfortable home, were safe, and were a family. Overnight, that all changed.

I lived in a small one-bedroom apartment, with no room for three children and a three-year-old granddaughter. I was picking up odd jobs to pay my way, and had about $800 when they called and asked to come and live with me. It was like buying the GMC Jimmy all over again; only this time things were kind of in reverse; my children were depending on their dad again like they always had. I didn't know how it was going work; I only knew I had to step into the dark and let faith work a miracle.

The kids arrived in June, 1989; and one blessing had already taken place. I found a nice home for rent in Orem, Utah, fully furnished, as the whole family was going to England for one year on a teaching assignment for the father. It was a four-bedroom home for six hundred and fifty dollars a month. When the children arrived, I had one hundred and fifty dollars to my name.

The first night they were in a comfortable home again; I know they all went to bed feeling safe and thought that everything would be normal again. I went to bed that first night not knowing what I was going to do; I just laid down and said, "Lord, this is all in your hands."

Desperate people do desperate things and my working at temporary jobs was not going to pay the rent, feed and clothe four children, or allow me to put things in place to the point where I could even think of continuing this crazy journey that I had started on five years earlier.

I wished that good people had not believed in what I was doing. Their money had produced successful therapies for people who had no hope for their skin disorders, and now I felt an obligation to continue, but had no idea how. Desperate, I went to the yellow pages in the phone book. In those pages I knew there was at least one person who could help, but how to find that person seemed almost an impossible task.

Instinctively, the first place I looked was under Financial Advisors. I picked out two at

Copyright 1996 Medisys Research Group, Inc.

random and called their offices for appointments. I met with both the next day. I gave them a history of everything that had been accomplished, and showed them the Ernst & Young audit along with Dr. MacGregor's report. To my surprise, both showed a genuine interest in my project and the first one asked me to return in a couple of days. But the second one, Dan Roberts, did not ask me to return. Mr. Roberts asked me one question. "How much did you receive for the last 1% equity in your company?" I told him approximately $90,000, but that my circumstances were such that I would take $30,000 for 1% equity. On the spot, he wrote me out a check for $10,000 and would have a check ready for $20,000 more when the proper agreements were completed.

Life is in fact stranger than fiction, because that $30,000 changed the course of medicine in the treatment of a broad range of serious to moderate skin diseases, not to mention the immediate need to care for my family.

Although I cannot elaborate for personal, but good reasons, Dan Roberts received his investment back several times over; but more important than money, I was able to return the favor in a way that neither of us could have ever imagined at the time of our first meeting. They say that coincidence is the principle upon which God remains anonymous. Oh how true!

Funding Adventure

The $30,000 from Dan Roberts also gave me valuable time needed to focus just on funding for research. I was introduced to a man in Utah who had a reputation for securing funds for worthy projects. After reviewing a business plan I had put together, he assured me that funding to the tune of $1 million would not be a problem. I gave him a copy of the business plan feeling optimistic about the future.

About eight months later, never hearing a word from the man, my phone rang. The person calling wanted to know if I knew so and so; and did I have any connection to a research project involving skin care. I said yes to both questions, and let him know that I had not seen or heard from the person he asked about for eight months. He then told me this man had secured large sums of money from him and some of his friends. He went on to tell me that some of the funds had been used to set up a skin care clinic, and the rest of the money he pocketed for himself. It was a scam, but one that turned in my favor.

I made arrangements to meet with the caller and his friends. I discovered that they and others had invested between $500,000 and $1 million. They then told me the location of the skin care clinic trying to use our therapies and trying to reproduce our exclusively formulated soaps and moisturizers. I couldn't believe someone could be that brazen and really dumb enough to think they could get away with it.

I asked the five men in the room where we met if one person in that room had even picked up the phone to do some due diligence and check out any of the names or places mentioned in the business plan they had been shown. Not one of them had done any due diligence. If they had, they would have discovered that the real names and places in the business plan did not exist; as the scammer had put in phony names and places. These investors had lost their money.

As a result of this meeting, I went to the Utah Division of Securities and Exchange and shared the information I had. They requested that I meet with them again. In the next meeting they had requested that the manager of the clinic be there which allowed them to get more detailed information. Come to find out, there was an investigation already taking place as a result of complaints from patients of the phony clinic because of side effects they were experiencing from the soaps and moisturizers they had tried to replicate at the clinic.

In the meeting, the clinic manager admitted that he knew something was wrong with the whole set-up at the clinic, and that he had the authority to turn over the clinic to me, lock, stock, and barrel if I would not pursue any criminal charges. This did not release the scam artist from charges that would be brought by the Utah Securities and Exchange Commission. The rumor passed on to me was that those charges were dropped in exchange for information on a much larger scam that the man was involved in in another state with other people.

Needless to say, I didn't care what happened to the scam artist; I now had ownership of a medical clinic, fully staffed, which made getting legitimate funds much easier, and opened up the doors to an opportunity I thought would be difficult to achieve, and much further down the road. We took the lemon and made lemonade! Dan Roberts believed in me, and I believed all things were possible. Little did I know how events could change things so quickly. Another helping hand, another miracle.

Patents

Way before the Gresham Medical Center Studies, I had filed for use patents on the topical medications that already had FDA approval for internal use. After three different patent firms had failed to secure the patent rights, I all but gave up. Then someone thought I ought to meet with Lynn Foster, a patent attorney in Salt Lake City who had a great reputation as a patent attorney. I met with Lynn, and he felt I had tried for so many years that even if he were successful, there would be little time left on a patent even if it were awarded. He felt that the only way it would have any value was if I abandoned the patent and re-filed a new patent. He said it was a gamble for two reasons. If someone else in the interim had filed a similar patent, I was out of luck; and if not, there was certainly no guarantee that he would succeed where three other patent attorneys had failed. I told him to abandon the patent and roll the dice. He did, and he was successful.

First Medical Clinic

Now that we had our first clinic, we were in a position to treat patients with cystic to moderate acne, and a broad range of eczema conditions. With a 90% success rate, no side effects, and a fee structure that allowed anyone with or without medical insurance to be treated, we were in business. But more importantly, we now had the resources to investigate many more skin diseases.

In a short time we were able to train more medical assistants which allowed us to open a second clinic in Provo, Utah, which had a large population of college students, and young men and women at the LDS Missionary Training Center.

Things were coming together faster than we anticipated, and the decision was made to open a third clinic in Pocatello, Idaho, a city of about fifty thousand people. This took place around 1997. Little did we know that the Pocatello Clinic would open the door to a treasure of information.

Copyright 1996 Medisys Research Group, Inc.

I went to the Pocatello Clinic every other week to meet with the clinic's physician and medical assistants. Fortuitism, luck, or whatever you want to call it, I was at the clinic when a mother and her eight-year-old daughter had come down from Montana to see if there was anything we could do for her daughter's psoriasis. The little girl was literally covered from head to foot with horrible patches of sores and flaking skin.

I was able to sit in the patient room while the doctor got her medical history. I had previous experiences where there were hints that we would one day learn enough about psoriasis to successfully treat the disease. Well, on this day, I learned what I needed to know to go for it.

The little girl's mother, in giving a history of her daughter's experience, explained that two years previous, her daughter had developed a sore on both of her knees. The sores were treated by both the parents and a physician for a full year with no success. Then, almost overnight, she had developed psoriasis over her entire body. When I heard this, it was like a light switched on. I was 99% sure what had happened, and learned more about psoriasis in sixty seconds than I had learned in all my years of research.

I suspected that this patient had scraped her knee, or something else had caused the sores to open up, and the infection had now entered into her blood, and provided the necessary conditions for the infection (psoriasis) to spread throughout her body, and produced the psoriasis patches over her body from head to foot.

Making this assumption, the patient's mother agreed to a new approach to treating her daughter. This meant that she had to stop going to the University of Utah Hospital for UV therapies and anything else that was being done to calm her psoriasis down. We wanted a "cure," and with some research on old and new broad-spectrum antibiotics, I settled on Lorabid, which for some reason is now off the market. I decided on ten days of Lorabid internally, and Doxycycline administered topically. This was done in conjunction with other requirements in the treatment protocol, all of which is disclosed in the section of this book concerning the treatment of many other skin disorders.

After 15 weeks of treatment, the eight-year-old psoriasis patient was completely free of psoriasis. This therapy has been repeated with other psoriasis patients with the same success.

MOLLUSCUM

Coincidence being the principle upon which God remains anonymous, again, by pure chance I made the trip to our Pocatello Clinic.

While spending the day there, a mother came in with her boy who was to my best recollection, about six years of age. I was able to sit in while the physician took the patient's history. He had previously been diagnosed with molluscum—a skin condition which I had not seen before. The symptoms are very specific and appear as raised, thin eruptions of skin that come in clusters just about anywhere on the body. This patient had been treated with no success, and the condition was spreading.

When I heard that the condition was spreading, that was all I needed to know to draw my own conclusions about the cause of this skin disorder. What was causing this skin disease to spread? The condition caused itching and scratching. After scratching, the young patient would touch other parts of his body which allowed the organisms from the skin eruptions to be spread to other parts of his body and start new clusters.

Treating this skin disease did not seem like rocket science. Little did I know that it was considered untreatable by the rest of the medical therapists. If I had known, I might have been a little intimidated by the challenge, but I was reasonably sure that we could develop a therapy that would succeed. Luckily, we were working with a mother who was willing to cooperate, and followed some of her own instincts while treating the boy with the protocol that had been developed. Thank God for her perseverance and staying the course. Her boy became symptom free, and today there is no reason for anyone to experience some of the horrible, dead-end therapies that are practiced even today without success on molluscum.

This therapy protocol will be disclosed in the chapter covering many other skin disorders.

The Theoretical Premise for Most Skin Disorders

I hesitate to use the word "theoretical" when it has been demonstrated thousands of times in clinical settings around the world that we got something right with a 90% success rate with a broad range of skin conditions. But I have learned after twenty-five years that there is much more to learn by those willing to dedicate their time and research to build on what I have learned. If others will carry on, I know for a certainty that their research will open doors for the successful treatment of other serious health problems; not the least being cancer. A silver bullet?...maybe.

What causes so many different symptoms that are characterized as skin disorders or more appropriately "skin diseases"?

The premise and conclusions will be lain out in terms and explanations in language that medical students, physicians, and laymen can all understand and apply, not only to the different treatment protocols included in this book, but will open the door for the treatment of most skin diseases.

Skin diseases are bacterial infections that result from a deficient immune system. That being the case, then why can't we just treat them with a simple course of a broad spectrum antibiotic? Well, many physicians try with some skin diseases with little or no success. Sometimes they do more harm than good.

Not knowing the cause and effect can generate confusion which results in so many wild and unorthodox attempts at treatment, they're not even worth discussing. They are as criminal and ineffectual as electric shock treatments and lobotomies performed on patients that are mentally ill.

To say there is a common denominator which exists and interferes with the patients' immune system would be misleading. But we will discuss some common factors that exist and will explain why a dose of antibiotics will not do the job on its own, but must be part of a treatment that goes on after all the contributing factors involved in a patient's skin condition are assessed. There is nothing more important, with no exceptions, than getting the most detailed patient history that you can.

Copyright 1996 Medisys Research Group, Inc.

The following outline of some common factors existing with a patient are only those that I have come to recognize over twenty-five years of research. My prediction is that some observant and bright student of skin diseases may find something common in the cause of most skin disorders.

Stress

Most cultures inherently produce some forms of stress...some more than others. In those cultures where competition is high; whether for money, recognition, status, safety, or food, etc., stress will be high. Is that to say then that everyone who has significant stress in their lives is going to experience a skin disorder? No, but in the United States approximately 20% or sixty million people experience some kind of skin disorder.

How about the other 80%? Stress affects different people in different ways—all the way from sleepless nights, some form of drug or alcohol addiction, heart problems, weakened immune systems, to cancer. Then there are those who have learned to handle their stress, get plenty of sleep, and hardly ever get sick. What is their secret? That is another whole book.

I, myself, having lived amongst the Navajo people in the southwestern United States for thirty months, learned firsthand the effects of living in a stress-free environment. I was twenty-one years old, and had just completed four years in the U.S. Air Force, with three of those years spent in Germany from 1954 to 1957. I had adult acne which caused me no small discomfort. After living with the Navajos for six months, my acne completely cleared up, and my skin became luxurious. I went to bed at night after a long day and discovered that morning seemed to come about ten minutes after I went to bed. There was no dreaming, and upon waking up I was fresh and wide awake. How true the saying, "I slept like a log."

I slept in the same sleeping bag for 30 months; bathed, washed my face, and shaved in water taken from the windmill tanks from which the horses and sheep drank. The water had no negative effect on my skin whatsoever, and I was sick a total of three days in thirty months, and at six feet two inches tall, I returned home to Portland, Oregon weighing one hundred and thirty-eight pounds.

After being home for thirty days, sleeping in fresh clean sheets and pillow cases, and bathing in clean tap water, my acne returned in full blossom, along with the stresses of everyday living.

Theory

My firm belief is that stress produces a chemical reaction in our systems—whether it's excess acid in our colon, excess adrenalin, hormones, or whatever, it has a profound effect on our whole immune system resulting in ill health in some form or another. The challenge is to discover what this chemical reaction is and neutralize it. Somebody will.

Copyright 1996 Medisys Research Group, Inc.

Sleep

In the meantime, what can we do to help reduce our stress levels? I could write a whole book on my views about stress, but let me give you the best one-liner I can on stress.

No matter how much you worry about any kind of event or problem in your life that causes stress, ninety-nine percent of the time the event or problem will end exactly the same whether you stress over it or not. The only exception is an event or problem for which you can do something to influence the end result. The solution is then simple: do something, but just don't do nothing, and make yourself sick stressing over it.

So, what can sleep do for stress? It calms your whole physiological system. Your brain needs to rest, and be free from worry. It is only in sleep that your whole body can heal and rejuvenate itself.

But you say, how can I sleep when I am stressed from worry? For sleep you will discover that there are many options which I will not get into. But I will disclose one that has worked for everyone I know personally. It is a prescription drug you may have already heard of. Zanax or the generic form called Alprazolam for anxiety. It is better than "any" sleeping pill I am aware of. (0.5 mg usually does the job.)

Is it addictive? Yes, depending on the person using the drug. I have used it for twenty years for sleep, and have no craving for it during the daytime. Am I addicted? I am addicted to sleep, and getting off Zanax would be a gradual process, and at seventy-five years old, I don't want to take the time to go through the process. If you have an addictive personality, and would rely on it to get through the day, I would suggest that you not use the drug unless your physician thinks it's a viable option.

In the end, no matter what option you choose, you need a good eight hours sleep a night to help you through the next day, but most important to help strengthen your immune system to assist in the therapy protocols you will use for your individual skin disorder.

Yeast

Most of us have yeast in our system, more specifically, our digestive system. When we get too much yeast, it impacts our body's chemistry and affects our body's immune system, therefore directly affecting our skin disorder.

What can we do to minimize our yeast overload? I could discuss different remedies at length, but for our purposes here I will disclose two directives that we insist on for patients whom we have treated over the years. Processed sugars of any origin—and for the first eight weeks of therapy, no natural sugars. Yeast thrives on sugars, and so we try to starve it out of existence. Patients will say they can't go through the withdrawal of sugar from their diet. We gently tell them that they are not a candidate for our therapies, and they will have to seek help from somewhere else. Getting off processed sugar is difficult for some patients, but they do it rather than live with their skin disorder.

In conclusion, with no sugar we have the patient get on a good probiotic such as Primadaphalis. These probiotics contain beneficial organisms necessary for a healthy digestive system. Because of so many prescription drugs, such as antibiotics, we destroy those naturally occurring organisms so necessary for our digestive system to function properly.

Copyright 1996 Medisys Research Group, Inc.

Processed sugars eliminated from your diet and the introduction of a good probiotic, are both necessary in the eradication of your skin disease. Until someone comes up with a magic pill, there are no shortcuts in treating these skin diseases.

Liver

Skin diseases for the most part are symptomatic of something gone wrong inside our physical bodies. Either we are neglecting something that has gone wrong, or we are introducing substances into our bodies that can cause great harm to the health of our organs, and/or our immune system.

One of the things we want a patient to concentrate on is their liver. An unhealthy liver can result in bad health affecting other organs and negative chemical reactions—all of which can result in serious skin disorders.

What can we do to rejuvenate our liver? Luckily our liver is the only organ in the body that can be rejuvenated. By this I mean, you can cut 80% of it off, and under the right conditions and help, the liver will grow back. How lucky can we be? Without your liver, you will die; it processes all the chemicals, good and bad, from things you put into your body. If you overwhelm the liver with bad chemicals, "poisons," you will destroy it. Just as the alcoholic that dies from cirrhosis of the liver.

The old saying, "You are what you eat," is so true. And nowadays, all in the name of money and greater profits, producers of food are deliberately poisoning our systems with both processed and sadly *unprocessed* foods. We can only do our best to search out the best and safest foods for our diet. Even though labels on processed foods can be misleading, at least read them and educate yourself on what is reasonably safe and healthy and will do the least amount of damage. Doing these things helps your liver to function with less effort, and helps promote overall good health.

Since most of us part of the time, and some of us all the time, put unhealthy substances into our bodies, we need to give our liver a helping hand. One way we have done this with our patients in conjunction with the things we have already discussed is to introduce them to a sixty-day supplement of "milk thistle extract." Two capsules per day is needed to clean your liver and help it to rejuvenate and function properly. I do a liver cleanse once a year.

I try to eat healthy, but unless you produce your own food, you are at the mercy of the local grocery store, and so a liver cleanse each year helps to give you an edge.

In the first three or four weeks you will probably notice a significant loss of energy, along with some diarrhea. This condition only tells you that the liver is responding, and in four weeks your energy will return stronger than when you started.

Vitamin C

For adults, a daily dose of 1000 mg in the morning and 1000 mg in the evening will compliment all the things you are doing, as well as add to healthy skin and a healthier life. Capsules are more easily absorbed. Children under 12 years old should take 1000 mg per day.

Copyright 1996 Medisys Research Group, Inc.

Testimonials

Dear American Institute of Skin Care,

About two years ago, I sat on a doctor's table remembering how in junior high through high school I'd considered myself lucky never to go through the pain and humiliation my friends did with their awful torturous medications and special diets in the war for a clear face. I was just elated that I was clear.

Really, I was just clearly late, and now I was desperately trying to get my old face back.

The doctor walked in and asked me what seemed to be my trouble. I sheepishly answered, "I keep getting zits." He just looked at me and with an amused shake of his head he told me sternly. "You have acne. Why are people so reluctant to say that?"

Because, to a nineteen-year-old already self-conscious adolescent, the word "acne" is equivalent to "the plague."

I left with a prescription and a list of soaps to try, and the half-hearted assurance, "you'll figure it out."

A year later I'd given up on looking my best. I'd stopped wearing makeup because the artist side of my brain said, "What's the use if you don't have a clean canvas to start with?"

On a whim I picked up the yellow pages and an ad caught my eye. "We succeed where others failed." Well, the others had failed. Hundreds of dollars worth of the latest prescription-strength medications hadn't given me the confidence I needed to stay dedicated through the very slow process of clearing up my skin.

You told me, up front, the changes in my daily routine I would need to make to clear me up once and for all. I could go on and on about how I didn't feel embarrassed once during my consultations with you or the fact that the visits themselves were exactly what I needed to stay on track until I could see improvements.

The bottom line—you do succeed where others fail, and I'm proud to say—your system is as flawless as my face.

Sincerely, Summer Gale

I am a 69-year-old Type II diabetic for the past 15 years.

The first of 2001 I was diagnosed with a deep ulcer on the bottom of my foot going to the bone. The doctor advised me to go to bed and stay off my foot for 10 days as she feared the infection would go so deep that the foot would have to be amputated.

Gary Heesch, President of Wasatch Pharmaceutical, heard about my problem and gave me a patented lotion manufactured by Wasatch Pharmaceutical to be applied several times during the day. I applied this lotion every day to the ulcer on my foot. When I returned to the doctor's office after 10 days the doctor was so surprised at the fact that the ulcer was completely healed that she called in two other doctors to look at the foot. She made the comment that she was shocked at how well the ulcer had healed and that she was anticipating infection in the bone and a possible amputation.

Jerry D. Timothy

Acne Treatment

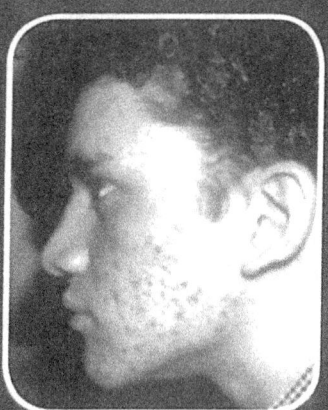
Before

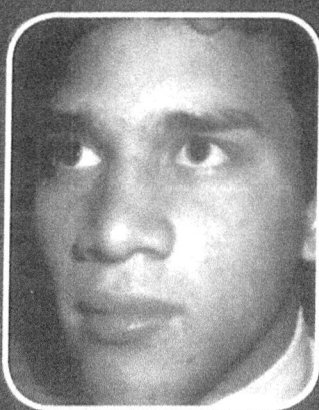
After

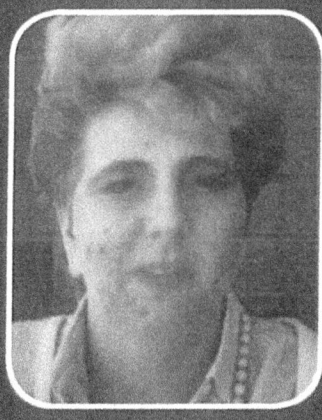
Before

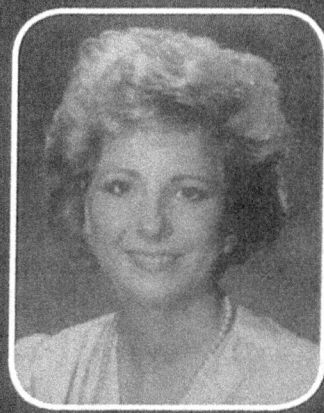
After

Psoriasis Treatment

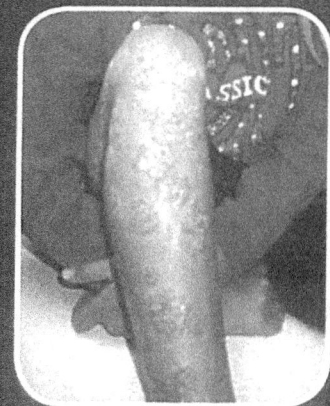
Before

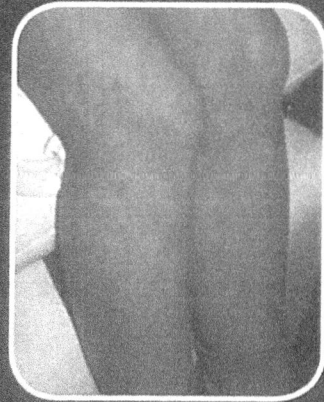
After

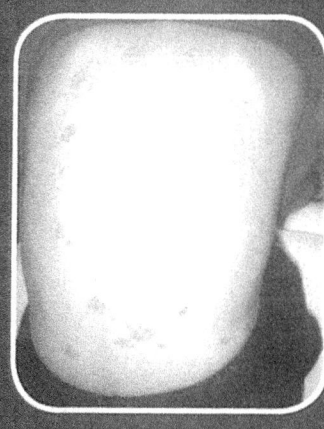
Before

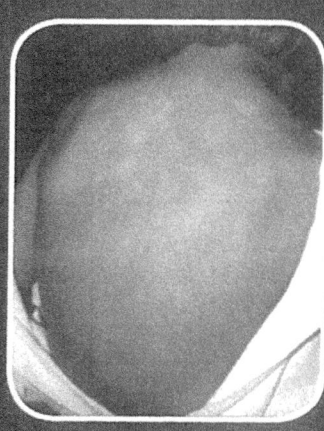
After

Eczema Treatment

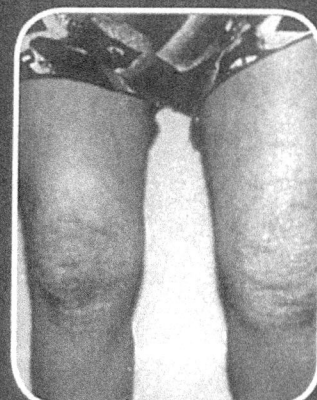
Before

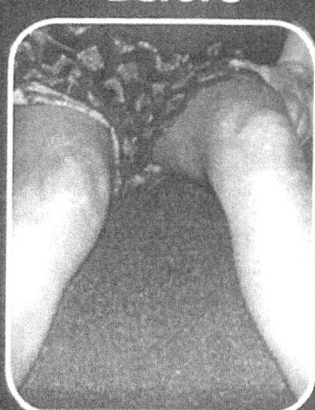
After

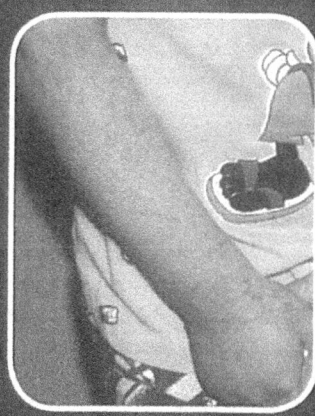
Before

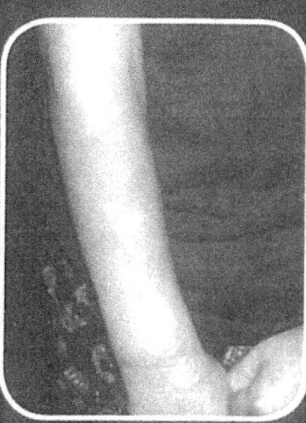
After

GRESHAM MEDICAL CENTER
Eczema Testing
Summary Report
For
Dermacare Pharmaceuticals

In late 1985 and early 1986, during the Chesebrough/Dermacare testing program for acne conducted at the Gresham Medical center, two patients having both acne and eczema found that their eczema conditions responded successfully to the same treatment being used to clear their acne condition. A third subject, a long-standing patient of the Center with chronic hand eczema was started on the eczema regime in January 1986 and her hands were completely cleared in two weeks.

As a consequence of these unexpected results, Dermacare Pharmaceuticals requested a follow-up study on eczema to determine the efficacy of its treatment on various conditions. Eleven eczema patients, ranging in age from five to 64 years old, participated in this eczema program in the Fall of 1986. Characteristics of the 14 eczema conditions treated at the Center in 1985-86 are outlined in the following paragraphs.

1. 13 out of the 14 patients experienced complete eradication of their symptoms.

2. One of the 14 patients did not respond to treatment.

3. One eight-year old female with a history of total body eczema from age six weeks recovered completely.

4. One 12-year old male patient with total body eczema from age six years recovered completely.

5. Six patients, children and adults with hand eczema over a period of several years, experienced complete recovery. Most of these were severe conditions.

6. Three patients with hand and arm eczema, two severe, recovered completely. These were children and adults.

7. Two patients, one male and one female, both adults, had a long history of face eczema, and both experienced complete recovery.

8. All patients in the study had an extensive history of medical attention without any significant results.

9. 12 of the 13 patients treated successfully experienced an eradication of their symptoms within 12 weeks. The one exception would have recovered within 12 weeks if instructions had been followed. Once the patient adhered to the program, her recovery was consistent with the rest of the test group.

10. This was a self-treatment program which took approximately five minutes per day in their home.

11. All patients concluded that the treatment procedures were easy to follow and that the therapy was without side effects.

CONCLUSIONS

The conclusions in this study are self-evident when one considers the ranges in ages, sex, and types of eczema conditions, and all having an extensive history of various medical treatments now available in the United States. The results of this test group are dramatic and conclusive. The active ingredient, and the methodology developed by Dermacare Pharmaceuticals is an effective and exciting therapy for a broad range of eczema conditions, and, will without doubt, become the drug of choice for the treatment of eczema.

Malcolm MacGregor, M.D.

June, 1987

Wasatch Business Plan Appendix

GRESHAM MEDICAL CENTER
Acne/Eczema Testing
for Dermacare Pharmaceuticals

Patient Summaries
June, 1987

Summary TJJ: This 23-year old WF was first seen 9/18/85 with a history of acne from age 11. She had used all known forms of treatment with little success. Although she had recurrent minor breakouts, she was very happy with the results until last seen on 1/29/86 when she declined to proceed. I consider her a failure although she should have been followed longer.

Summary BEM: This 20-year old WM first seen on 11/21/85. He was very introverted probably due to his severe acne. When last seen on 3/6/86 he was almost clear and very happy. He did not return for follow-up.

Summary JRM: This 14-year old WM, a regular patient, was first started on the regime for acne on 11/18/85. He was always an uncooperative patient and his folloing of the regime was questionable but when seen for other problems on 3/24/86 his acne was cleared. This is a case of a good result depite poor patient cooperation.

Summary KLH: This 28-year old WF first seen on 11/2/85 with cystic mild facial acne heretofore resistant to treatment. On the regime, she was clear within four weeks and remained so for the 12-week follow-up period.

Summary DVT: This 21-year old oriental male first seen on 11/5/85 with severe cystic acne. He was eager for treatment and his results were excellent. He was all clear in one month. He did have a breakout later and was advised to change his living habits as well.

Summary PLR: This 22-year old WM first seen on 12/30/85 with moderately severe acne. He did improve and when last seen on 6/7/86 had no pustules. This is an example of a case that will need prolonged use of the regime.

Summary BWH: This 16-year old WM first seen 8/12/85 with severe corporal and mild facial acne. He did not follow the regime well and had frequent NSOV. Started over because of this on 1/2/86. When seen on 9/6/86 for another problem, he was free of facial acne. This is a case that proves that the patient must be cooperative for a good result.

Summary JAS: This 15-year old WM first seen on 11/19/85 for severe facial acne with prolific comedones. On 1/2/86, his face was clear. An excellent result.

Wasatch Business Plan Appendix

Summary DGN: This 14-year old WM with severe facial acne first seen on 1/29/86. He was cleared by the 10th week. An excellent result.

Summary WWC: This 16-year old WM was first seen 11/16/85 with severe facial acne treated for two years with poor results. He cleared by the 16th week. An excellent result.

Summary TRT: This 17-year old WM first seen 11/16/85 with five-year history of facial acne. By the 4th week of the regime, he was almost clear and feeling good about the results. He had a mild breakout on the 12th week when he went off the program for one week.

Summary NJA: This 23-year old WM first seen 1/31/86 with a nine-year history of facial acne. This would be classified as cystic acne on his neck region. He was completely clear on the 12th week of the regime.

Summary DMR: This 29-year old WF first seen on 9/10/86 with chronic, pruritic eczema of the hands. This problem covers seven years with occasional acute blistering. By week two, she was completely healed. When last seen on 11/26/86, she was still disease free and ecstatic about the results.

Summary DJG: This 17-year old WM was first seen 9/24/86 with severe chronic eczema of his palms and wrists. Soles of his feet were also involved. When last seen on 11/26/86, he was completely healed.

Summary DG: This 42-year old WF first seen on 9/24/86 with mild chronic hand eczema. When last seen on 11/26/86, she had eczema on her right index finger only. It should be noted that she was stressed due to a one-month old daughter.

Summary CAW: This 36-year WF, long-standing patient, started on eczema regime on 1/28/86 for chronic hand eczema. Within two weeks, her hands were all clear. She has been on the regime since the above date and is perfectly controlled.

Summary ERG: This 3-year old WM started on the regime 9/24/86 for eczema of his thumbs and eyelids. Was all clear on 10/22/86 and remained so when last seen on 11/26/86.

Summary JG: This 9-year old WM started on regime 9/24/86 for excoriated eczema of his arms and elbows. When last seen on 12/3/86 was much improved.

Summary BJR: This 8-year old WF started on the regime for eczema on 9/11/86. This eczema was chronic and involved her trunk, buttocks, legs, and arms. This was a very resistant and severe eczema, chronic since age six months. Results were amazing in that she was completely cleared of her eczema on 3/14/87.

Summary WER: This 19-year old WM was first seen on 2/8/86 for moderately severe facial acne of four years duration. He cleared completely by the 6th week.

Summary SMB: This 32-year old WF first seen on 10/24/85 with cystic facial acne. Improved by week eight and cleared completely by 1/9/86.

Summary BSS: This 33-year old BF with severe cystic acne was started on the program 10/4/85. She cleared well by the 10th week except for permanent scarring.

Summary CFM: This 20-year old WM started on the program 9/19/85 for moderately severe facial acne. Although he was not faithfully following instructions and frequently missed office visits he cleared well by 1/21/86.

Summary JWS: This 33-year old WM with mild recurrent facial acne on 9/18/85 was started on the regime. He was all clear on 12/19/85 and remained clear when last seen on 1/6/86. His intention was to remain on the program.

Summary JMF: This 21-year old WM with moderately severe facial acne consisting of numerous comedones, papules and pustules was started on the regime on 11/8/85. He cleared by the 12th week then went off the program for 3-4 weeks and had another breakout. He was back on the program and doing well when last seen on 4/19/86.

Summary KJP: This 25-year old WF with chronic hand eczema and mild facial acne was started on both regimes on 12/3/85. Both problems were all cleared by the 2nd week.

Summary BKS: This 33-year old with mild acne was started on the regime on 3/18/86. She cleared well by the 2nd week and remained so for the 12-week session.

Summary ST: This 16-year old WF started on the regime 2/13/86 for moderate facial acne. She cleared by the 4th week. She was very happy with the program when last seen on 4/22/86.

Summary GWC: This 16-year old WM with mild facial acne started on the regime 1/30/86. He was improved by the 2nd week and completely clear by the 4th week and remained so through the 10th week.

Summary DTB: This 16-year old WM with mild facial acne started on the regime 1/30/86. He was improved by the 2nd week and completely clear by the 4th week and remained so through the 10th week.

Summary MT: This 27-year old WM with moderately severe facial acne started the regime 10/19/85. He was all cleared by the 10th week on 12/28/85. When seen on 2/8/86 after going off the program he had a recurrence and was started back on the medication.

Summary JML: This 21-year old WF with moderately severe acne, mostly comedones and papules, started the regime 2/5/86. She was almost clear by the 4th week, cleared completely on the 8th week, and remained so through week 12.

Summary WMC: This 22-year old WF with moderate facial acne started the regime 1/29/86. In the 3rd week, she was not faithful to the program and flared after a second week marked improvement. She cleared completely week 12 in spite of this early set back.

Summary ER: This 64-year old WF with recurrent facial pyoderma was started on the regime 9/10/86. She was cleared within a week and remained so when last seen on 10/28/86.

Summary CJW: This 32-year WF with chronic hand and wrist eczema of six years duration was started on the regime 9/19/86. She cleared completely by 11/8/86.

Summary JAS: This 31-year old WM with chronic atopic eczema of his hands, wrists, and knees was started on the regime 9/17/86. He may have reacted to the medication and went off the program on 10/8/86. Treatment of this patient is considered to be unsuccessful.

Summary CMP: This 12-year old WM with severe chronic eczema involving his hands, nail beds, forearms, forehead, body and elbows started the regime 9/10/86. He responded almost immediately and was clearing well by 9/27/86. He was completely clear on 11/26/86.

Summary PB: This 22-year old white female with severe psoriasis of her elbows was started on the program on 9/10/86. When last seen on 10/9/86, the rash was improved and the puritus was totally gone.

Summary WP: This 30-year old white male with moderate acne and moderately severe facial eczema was started on the program in January 1986, and within sex weeks was cleared of both his acne and eczema condition.

Malcolm Macgregor, M.D.

CURRICULUM VITAE
Malcolm D. Macgregor, M.D.

PERSONAL INFORMATION

Business Address:	Gresham Medical Center 495 NE Beech Street Gresham, Oregon 97030 Phone: 503-760-1433
Date of Birth:	December 9, 1925 Eugene, Oregon
Social Security No:	543-20-9331

EDUCATION

High School:	Eugene High School Eugene, Oregon	1939-43
Undergraduate Education:	B.A., University of Oregon Eugene, Oregon	1946-50
Medical Education:	M.D., University of Oregon Portland, Oregon	1949-53

TRAINING SUBSEQUENT TO GRADUATION FROM MEDICAL SCHOOL

Internship:	University of Washington
	  Harborview Hospital
	  Seattle, Washington

Fellowship:	American Academy of Family Practice
	  Kansas City, Missouri
	American Academy of Cosmetic Surgery
	  Los Angeles, California
	Dermatology Institute of Miami
	  Miami, Florida

HONORS AND AWARDS

High School:	Member National Honor Society	1939-43
	President Senior Class	1943
	King of the Mardi Gras	
	French Speaking Club	1942
Undergraduate Education:	Friars Honorary	1949
	King of Hearts	1948
	President of Junior Class U. of O.	1949
	Lambda Chi Alpha	1947-50

APPOINTMENTS AND HONORS

Chairman of the Board Mt. Hood Community College	1980
Chairman of "Quit Smoking Clinic" American Cancer Society	1968
Chief of Staff Gresham Community Hospital	1960

COMMUNITY SERVICE

Gresham Historical Society
 Lifetime Member
School Boards – 10 Years Service
Chairman Elementary School Board   1968
Established Medical Assistants
 Program at Mt. Hood Community
 College
Class Instructor Medical Assistants
 Program

PRIVATE PRACTICE OF MEDICINE

Family Practice:

Gresham, Oregon   1955-87
Member Portland Academy of
 Hypnosis   1964-87
Served as classroom instructor
 and public awareness programs
 on medical hypnosis.
Member American Academy of
 Family Practice   1956-87

RESEARCH

Studied effect of Selenium and
 Vitamin E on White Muscle
 Disease in cattle.   1959-60
Clinical use of intravenous
 Vitamin C for viral infections
 and allergies.   1967-87
Clinical use of Nutri-wheat in
 lowering serum lipids including
 conferences on human nutrition
 with Dr. Arnold Spicer.   1984-87
Clinical trials with Gary
 Heesch's acne program.   1985-87

MILITARY SERVICE

U.S. Army

Infantry Staff Sergeant, WW2
Bronze Star, Purple Heart

Wasatch Business Plan Appendix

Ernst & Young

317 Sixth Avenue, Suite 1100
Des Moines, Iowa 50309

Telephone (515) 243-2727

REPORT ON EXAMINATION OF MEDICAL RECORDS

Medisys Research Group, Inc.
    And
Medisys of Iowa, Inc.

We have examined the medical records of selected patients treated with the Dermacare Treatment for acne and eczema to determine whether the records indicate the results of the treatment were successful. Our examination was made in accordance with standards established by the American Institute of Certified Public Accountants and included such procedures as we considered necessary in the circumstances.

We examined the medical records of twenty-eight patients selected from a population of thirty-nine patients in a research study group and ten patients in a preclinical test group. In addition, we interviewed fifteen of these patients or a parent to further support results of the treatment as documented in the medical records.

Because we are not licensed in the practice of medicine and do not purport to be experts in the practice thereof, we are unable to and do not express any opinion as to the effectiveness of the Dermacare Treatment for acne and eczema. In our opinion, the medical records examined for the twenty-eight patients selected from the aforementioned research study group and preclinical test group indicate the overall results of their treatment were successful.

Ernst & Young

December 12, 1989

Wasatch Business Plan Appendix

Ernst & Young

150 South Wacker Drive
Chicago, Illinois 60606

Telephone (312) 368-1800

December 12, 1989

Gary Heesch
Gresham Medical Center
495 Northeast Beach Street
Gresham, Oregon 97030

Dear Mr. Heesch:

We have completed our case review for Gresham Medical Center. Our review included a visit to your office, interviews with selected patients, and review of medical records.

The purpose of the review was to evaluate the overall treatment results for acne and eczema patients treated at the Gresham Medical Center. The scope of the review was to determine that the medical records indeed documented the efficacy of the treatment protocol, administration of the treatment, and documented treatment results, verified by patient interviews.

Our findings are included on the following pages.

It has been a pleasure serving the Gresham Medical Center and we appreciate the time you and your staff spent with us during this engagement. If you have any questions regarding this report or any other aspect of our services, please feel free to call Jean Mosebach at (312) 606-2385.

Very truly yours,

Ernst + Young

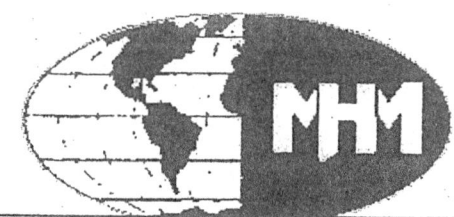

M-H MEDISCO, INC.

June 26, 1993

Gary V. Heesch, President
Medisys Research Group
714 East Ft. Union Blvd.
Midvale, Utah 84047

Dear Mr. Heesch;

In response to your request that we keep you informed as to our progress in the marketing of Medisys Research Group's technology and products I will summarize our basic agreement as well as the results of our efforts.

Under the option agreements, M-H Medisco secured the rights to conduct test marketing of products developed by Medisys Research Group for the treatment of two serious skin diseases, acne, including cystic acne, and eczema. It was agreed that if test marketing proved to be successful, M-H Medisco reserved the rights to exercise its option for a permanent agreement.

We have achieved the objectives of our test-marketing program and the results are as follows:

1. Total number of Physicians involved: 242

2. Total number of patients treated for acne and eczema: Approximately 2,000

3. Patient response to therapy for acne. In those cases where patients kept scheduled appointments and followed regimen (approximately 85% of the patients completed treatment), in excess of 90% experienced successful treatment.

    Success is being interpreted as total or near total clearing of all symptoms with prevention of most reoccurring symptoms.

    These results were comparable to those achieved in the Medisys/Chesebrough studies conducted at the Gresham Medical Center in Gresham, Oregon.

P.O. BOX 211418 • SALT LAKE CITY • UTAH • 84121-8417
(801) 943-0335 • FAX (801) 943-0335

Gary V. Heesch, Medisys Research Group
Page 2

4. Patient response to therapy for eczema. In those cases where patients kept scheduled appointments and followed regimen (approximately 85% cooperated and followed instructions), in excess of 85% experienced successful treatment.

Success is interpreted as total or near total clearing of all symptoms in a broad range of eczema conditions and prevention of most reoccurring symptoms.

Again, these results were comparable to those achieved in the Medisys/Chesebrough studies conducted at the Gresham Medical Center in Gresham, Oregon.

Based on the results of these studies, M-H Medisco, in April, 1993, exercised their option agreement with Medisys, and entered into a distribution agreement which also allows them the non-exclusive right to market Medisys Medical Technologies and products to existing medical clinics throughout the United States and Canada.

Even though the test marketing results were extremely positive, just as important was the acceptance by physician and patient to the Medisys therapy. If our experience remains consistent throughout the remainder of our marketing schedule and if we can persuade the physicians to carry these products, we should easily achieve all of our goals, which is to insure the distribution of the Medisys products throughout the United States and Canada over the next five years.

We appreciate your support in both time and advise as we work with these physicians and look forward to a long and mutually profitable relationship.

Sincerely,

/s/ V. Lee Maxwell
V. Lee Maxwell, President

Comments

As you try to digest the things you have read, and study the therapy protocols, the extra time it takes per day usually adds up to ten minutes a day. So don't feel overwhelmed by what you have learned, but remember one thing. You will not eradicate your skin disorder if you do not follow the protocol for your condition. For those of you who feel that your condition is not discussed in any of the protocols, follow the protocol outlined for psoriasis, and if it is a serious condition, add an anti-fungal compound to the therapy.

The following therapy protocols are listed with the hope that you have finally found a solution to your problem. If you choose to involve your physician, and he or she wishes to discuss your condition with us, they may do so by calling 801-491-0177 for Medisys Research, and ask for Gary Heesch.

PSORIASIS

The premise for psoriasis and its treatment is that it falls into a class of skin diseases that are caused by a bacterial infection. Psoriasis differs from most other skin infections because it can be spread through the blood. Why it can affect just certain areas of the body or affect a person from head to foot is not a question that we have found an answer to yet, and maybe never will.

Because it can spread internally, it requires a treatment protocol that treats the patient both internally and topically. And like strep throat or pneumonia, the goal is to eradicate 100% of the infectious bacteria. Is that possible? Yes, but because the patient has demonstrated their susceptibility to the organism, I have included in the treatment protocol certain immune-boosting steps to help prevent its reoccurrence.

When treating psoriasis, years of experience have demonstrated no negative side effects of any kind. This is important to know because if there are any negative side effects, treatment should be stopped to examine their cause, such as sensitivity to any part of the protocol.

Psoriasis, like most of the skin diseases has its own timetable and set of healing steps it goes through. Within two to three weeks flaking should be dramatically reduced. In another two to three weeks hard patches of skin should start to fall off, revealing brand new pinkish-red, almost transparent-looking skin. Because that's what it is—new skin which in time will thicken and eventually blend in color with surrounding skin. When this happens, you continue to treat until there are no more signs of psoriasis—at which time you continue treating until the new skin thickens up and feels normal to the touch.

If the patient does not respond to the treatment, a patch test should be taken, and skin cells from the affected area should be sent to the lab to determine if another antibiotic needs to be substituted. There can be more than one kind of organism involved. If you do not follow the treatment protocol, you will not succeed in eradicating the skin disorder.

Copyright 1996 Medisys Research Group, Inc.

Don't Give Up, You Have Found Us 14

Psoriasis Protocol

Psoriasis is considered one of the more serious and hard to treat skin diseases. It is usually identified by such symptoms as inflammation of the skin, itching, and constant flaking of the skin followed by new skin cells. Psoriasis can stay confined to one area of the person's body or it can cover a person's body from head to foot; sometimes causing secondary infections that may become serious in and of themselves.

Our therapy for treating psoriasis is extremely successful if the patient is willing and committed to being symptom free and following the treatment schedule that is provided by *Medisys Research Group, Inc.* If not, we strongly suggest that you look elsewhere for a solution to your problem, as we cannot do you any good unless you are committed to following our protocol which has been successful with children and adults.

Treatment Schedule

Morning: Using a mild, fragrance free, and antibacterial free liquid soap; wash your hands and rinse thoroughly. Using the same soap, wash the affected area of the skin and let air dry or dry with a clean soft paper towel. Next, apply the liquid medication to the affected area and rub in thoroughly, then let air dry.

Mid-day: Apply liquid medication again.

Night: Shower or bathe every night with the liquid soap. After showering, do not dry the affected area with a cloth towel; let area air dry or use a paper towel, so as not to re-infect the skin.

Medication: *Eight of the medicine tablets (Doxycycline), should be put into four (4) oz. liquid containers. Allow three (3) hours for the tablets to dissolve at room temperature; keep medication refrigerated when not in use. Always shake bottles well before using. The powder in two capsules of Cefdinir, 300 mg, may be substituted for Doxycycline. Distilled water is used to put in the 4 oz. bottles.

Internal Medication: For ten (10) days, you will take 300 mg of Cefdinir three times a day.

- Milk thistle extract capsules – one taken in AM and one in PM for six weeks.

- Take 1 probiotic per day and 1,000 mg Vitamin "C" twice a day.

- At the end of your fourth week of treatment, you may purchase a mild, fragrance-free skin moisturizer and apply morning and night after your topical medication has thoroughly dried.

- In most cases, allow 12 to 15 weeks for your psoriasis to clear. Continue with the therapy another six (6) weeks after cleared of symptoms.

- When skin flaking has stopped and your skin in the affected area appears bright red or pinkish, it will over a period of weeks start to blend in color with the rest of your skin.

- No direct sunlight for five (5) months, exceeding 10 minutes a day.

Copyright 1996 Medisys Research Group, Inc.

- During this treatment schedule, you should not experience any adverse side effects. If you do, it means that you have sensitivity to one of the products you are using. If this happens, stop the use of all products and call 801-491-0177 so that we can evaluate and make any needed modifications in your therapy.

NOTE: Eat no processed or natural sugar for ten weeks. The absence of sugar in your diet and cleansing for most patients will result in ten to fifteen pounds of weight loss at the end of ninety days.

MOLLUSCUM

While visiting with a well-known dermatologist from the University in Colon, Germany in the year 2000, we were having lunch when he asked if I had worked with patients having Molluscum. I replied "Yes, but only a few." I told him our success rate was 100% and there was no reason to believe that would ever change. He was more than surprised, and I think a little bit disbelieving, and said that I would be a millionaire!

Well, I am not a millionaire, but have been rewarded many times over by the success I have observed with so many patients whose lives have returned to normal.

Molluscum is so mistreated by so many physicians with no success; it's difficult to comprehend their logic. Molluscum is actually a very straight forward skin disease to treat. Its symptoms are easy to recognize and can be found in clusters of raised, thin, lumps of skin with inflammation from scratching and spreading. It is not confined to any one area of the body and is caused from bacteria which can be spread by the patient's own fingers when scratching other parts of the body. It is usually brought under control within two weeks and eradicated in six weeks no matter how extensive it is over the body.

Where the infection comes from, how it starts, and why it exhibits the peculiar symptoms it does, I don't know. It's a peculiarity to the organism that causes it. It is a skin disease that deserves more investigation which I believe would lead to more interesting discoveries. For now, it's a comfort to know there is a cure as long as the treatment protocol is followed by the patient, and not modified by some practitioner.

Molluscum Protocol

Small, vertical, thin growths of skin or eruptions are symptomatic of Molluscum and will usually spread and can be found on different parts of the body. Molluscum can be found on children as well as adults. If not treated properly, the condition may cause secondary infections.

Treatment Schedule

Morning: Wash affected area with a clear, liquid soap that is fragrance free and _not_ an anti-bacterial. Before rinsing, use a <u>clean</u> washcloth, <u>rub</u> affected area after one week <u>vigorously</u>, and then rinse with clean water thoroughly. There will be some bleeding which is expected as the skin eruptions are rubbed off.

Copyright 1996 Medisys Research Group, Inc.

After rinsing thoroughly, let the affected area air dry or pat dry with a soft, clean paper towel. When skin is completely dry, spray on medication and rub in gently. When done, let skin air dry. Once dry, make sure clothing that touches affected areas is clean – this is VERY IMPORTANT.

Mid-day: Reapply medication only. Spray on and rub into affected area. Let air dry.

Night: Repeat morning routine.

Medication: *Eight (8) of the medicine tablets (Doxycycline), should be put into four (4) oz. liquid containers. Allow three (3) hours for the tablets to dissolve at room temperature; keep medication refrigerated when not in use. Always shake bottles well before using. Powder from two capsules of Cefdinir, 300 mg each, may be substituted for Doxycycline. Distilled water is used to fill the 4 oz. bottles.

IMPORTANT:

- Once skin is free of vertical eruptions; no longer rub area with a washcloth. Just gently wash and rinse area, and when skin is dry, spray on medication, gently rub in and let air dry. Allow 12 weeks to completely heal.

- Once dry, make sure clothing that touches affected areas is clean – this is VERY IMPORTANT.

- "Vitamin C": 12 years and under – 1,000 mg per day; 13 years and older – 2,000 per day.

- Eat no processed or natural sugar for ten (10) weeks. This is necessary to reduce yeast in digestive system.

- Drink at least four (4) glasses of water per day.

- Take one milk thistle extract capsule AM and PM each day for six (6) weeks to cleanse liver. You may experience diarrhea in the first two weeks and some loss of energy.

- Take a good probiotic each day.

- Drink no alcohol for the first ten (10) weeks.

CYSTIC ACNE / ACNE

With thousands of patients treated, the success rate for total eradication is 90% plus. Failures are for a variety of reasons, but generally can be attributed to the patients' lack of consistency in following the treatment protocol.

The treatment for cystic acne is often associated with the drug Acutane which destroys the oil glands with the premise that the oil produced has something to do with causing acne. Wrong.

Copyright 1996 Medisys Research Group, Inc.

Acutane can clear cases of cystic acne at great risk to the patient if they should experience any of the many side effects listed on the information provided to patients. The only reason Acutane can work is the fact that it restricts the release of a chemical excreted through the sebaceous glands that neutralizes the skin's inherent ability to fight the infection causing Acne. Oil from the sebaceous glands does help to provide a breeding ground for bacteria. There are many acne patients that have very dry skin. So there goes the theory for oil being the culprit.

The treatment protocol I have worked with for twenty-five years, along with the protocols for all the skin disorders I have treated, have produced no side effects of any consequence, and with cystic acne and less serious conditions of acne, our treatment protocol clears cystic acne in half the time as Acutane for a fourth of the cost - with no side effects.

Probably two of the primary causes of acne are stress, and diet. Our protocol deals with both of these issues along with providing a substitute for the patient's own immune system. In most cases, once the acne has cleared, it does not return.

Acne Treatment Protocol

For over twenty years, we have been treating a broad spectrum of skin diseases with medical therapies with virtually no side effects of any consequence. In treating cystic acne and lesser grades of acne, we have experienced a success rate in excess of 90% after treating thousands of patients.

With patents and copyrights in place and using FDA approved products, you will finally have a solution to your problem with the benefits of rejuvenated skin cells that give your skin a beautiful, luxurious appearance.

Because acne is a skin disease, our medical therapies are not a quick fix as you have often seen advertised on television and elsewhere. Our therapies provide a substitute for your own bodies' immune systems. In our years of experience, our treatment eradicates acne, cystic, or otherwise in 90% of patients treated. Your own immune system is able to work now and keep you free of acne and therefore prevent any reoccurrence.

In treating any disease, there is always one obstacle to a patient's success, and that is usually the patients themselves. If a patient is not committed to following the suggested protocol, then success will probably not be truly experienced. <u>For young girls or older women using our treatment protocols; if you use cover-up cosmetics on your face, you will not be successful with our therapies as you will only re-infect your skin</u>. Allow 8-12 weeks for your acne to clear, and be aware that in most cases your acne will get worse in the second or third week. This is normal. By the 5th or 6th week you will start to see improvement. After your acne has cleared, we recommend using the treatment schedule another six (6) weeks to prevent any reoccurrence.

Treatment Schedule

Morning: Wash hands with a clear liquid soap that is not antibacterial, and is fragrance free. Then wash face and other affected areas with the same soap. Men: use the same soap for shaving. Let face air dry or use a soft paper towel. Never use

Copyright 1996 Medisys Research Group, Inc.

a cloth towel to dry face or other affected areas as you will only re-infect your skin.

Once washed area has air-dried, apply medication (Doxycycline) in liquid bottles by spraying on affected areas and rub into the skin thoroughly with fingers and let air dry. Always shake bottle before using.

*Eight (8) of the medicine (Doxycycline) tablets should be put into four (4) oz. liquid containers. Allow three (3) hours for the tablets to dissolve at room temperature; keep medication refrigerated when not in use. Always shake bottles well before using. Powder from two capsules of Cefdinir, 300 mg each, may be substituted for Doxycycline. Distilled water is used to fill the 4 oz. bottles.

Day: If face gets sweaty or oily during daytime, use clean paper towels to pat face.

Night: Shower, wash hair, and repeat morning schedule. Do not put hairspray on at night.

IMPORTANT:

- Eat no sugar, processed or natural, nor drink alcohol for ten (10) weeks. This is done to clear the excess yeast from your body.

- Take a probiotic every day to help your digestive system and decrease yeast build-up.

- "Vitamin C: 12 years and under – 1,000 mg per day; 13 years and older – 2,000 mg per day.

- One milk thistle extract capsule should be taken twice a day – AM and PM for six (6) weeks.

- Change your pillow case(s) three (3) times a week.

- Once dry, make sure clothing that touches affected areas is clean – this is VERY IMPORTANT.

- Whiteheads on your skin: Rinse a straight pin under hot water and use gently to puncture the whitehead, and gently squeeze out white puss.

NOTE: The absence of sugar in the diet and cleansing for most patients will result in a ten to fifteen pound weight loss over ninety days.

ROSACEA

The treatment Protocol for Rosacea is not much different than that for acne. My experience with Rosacea patients has led me to believe that the root causes for Rosacea are stress, lack of adequate sleep which leads to a stronger susceptibility to contagions in the patient's environment, especially the workplace. Many physicians will treat their patients with a short and sometimes a long daily use of an antibiotic such as Minnocycline or Doxycycline,

Copyright 1996 Medisys Research Group, Inc.

which will help until the patient gets off the antibiotic; then back comes the Rosacea along with side effects from using the prescribed drug.

The treatment in our protocol is designed for a permanent solution with no side effects. This can be achieved if the patient is committed to ten minutes a day for ninety days in following the protocol as outlined for Acne.

FOLLICULITIS

This skin disorder is associated with hair follicles anywhere on the body and persons of all ages. It is an infection and is most common among African American males in their facial hairs as a result of shaving because of the facial hair's tendency to curl beneath the skin.

This skin disorder is treated much the same as acne; and for men shaving there will be instructions on how to keep the problem from reoccurring once the patient has cleared.

Folliculitis Protocol

Folliculitis is a skin disorder which causes body hair or whiskers to grow under the skin, causing mild to serious infections which only get worse with time if not treated properly. Our treatment is not a quick fix. We provide a substitute for your own immune system which eradicates the problem and allows your own immune system to keep you free of this skin disorder. Not only will this system eradicate your Folliculitis, but it will also rejuvenate your skin cells to give you clear, new-looking skin. Allow 8 to 12 weeks for clearing depending on the severity of your condition.

Treatment Schedule

Morning: Wash hands and face with a clear liquid soap that is not antibacterial, and is fragrance free.

If shaving, use the same liquid soap to lather your face that you use for shaving; rinse face thoroughly with warm water when finished shaving. Let face air dry or use a clean paper towel. Under no circumstances, use a cloth towel to dry your face or skin, as it will only re-infect your skin.
When your face is dry, apply the medication by spraying a small amount directly to the affected area two (2) or three (3) times and rub over your face thoroughly, then let it air dry.

Night: Except for shaving, repeat the same morning routine.

Medication: *Eight (8) of the medicine tablets (Doxycycline), should be put into four (4) oz. liquid containers. Allow three (3) hours for the tablets to dissolve at room temperature; keep medication refrigerated when not in use. Always shake bottles well before using. The powder in two capsules of Cefdinir, 300 mg, may be substituted for Doxycycline. Distilled water is used to fill the 4 oz. bottles.

IMPORTANT:

Copyright 1996 Medisys Research Group, Inc.

- Change your pillowcase three (3) times a week.

- Always shave downward to help prevent hairs from curling underneath the skin.

- Once dry, make sure clothing that touches affected areas is clean – this is VERY IMPORTANT.

- Eat no sugar, processed or natural, for ten (10) weeks. This is done to clear the excess yeast from your body.

- "Vitamin C": 12 years and under – 1,000 mg per day; 13 years and older – 2,000 per day.

- Take a milk thistle extract capsule twice a day – AM and PM for six weeks.

- Drink no alcohol for the first ten (10) weeks.

- Take a probiotic each day to help your digestive system and decrease yeast build-up.

- During the day, pat your face with a clean paper towel to get rid of excess oil. If you shower during the day, always reapply the medication.

NOTE: The absence of sugar in the diet and cleansing for most patients will result in a ten to fifteen pound weight loss over ninety days.

ATHLETE'S FOOT

Chronic Athlete's Foot can become quite serious. The standard treatment is on over-the-counter antifungal compound and/or a prescription antifungal drug. They can work temporarily, but more often than not the problem returns.

Why does it return and become worse? Simple; because the antifungal treatment does not get rid of the secondary infection which is bacterial. When the foot clears up, the remaining bacteria are left to grow and fester under the skin until finally the skin breaks open, the patient comes in contact with exposed fungus, and the patient is right back where they started.

Treating both causes of athlete's foot is only part of the protocol if the patient wants to remain free of reoccurring problems. So follow the protocol.

Athlete's Foot Protocol

Most cases of Athlete's Foot are chronic. In other words, a person treats Athlete's Foot with an over-the-counter anti-fungal treatment that clears up their Athlete's Foot, but more often than not, it returns even though some products say their product is a "cure." A cure should mean that the Athlete's Foot does not reoccur unless you puncture the skin on your foot and get

Copyright 1996 Medisys Research Group, Inc.

a new infection. With this protocol, you can expect your condition to clear within 8 to 12 weeks and not reoccur.

Treatment Schedule

<u>Morning</u>:

- Wash feet with a clear liquid soap.
- Dry with a paper towel.
- Spray on an over-the-counter anti-fungal spray.
- Let air dry.
- Spray on medication and let air dry.

<u>Mid-day</u>:

- Spray on medication.

<u>Night</u>:

- Repeat morning therapy.
- Wear clean socks each day - VERY IMPORTANT
- Eat no processed sugar for ten (10) weeks in order to reduce yeast build-up in digestive system.
- Take a probiotic every day for ten (10) weeks to help reduce yeast.
- Take a milk thistle extract capsule twice a day – AM and PM for six weeks.

Mixing Medication

*Eight (8) of the medicine tablets (Doxycycline) should be put into four (4) oz. liquid containers. Allow three (3) hours for the tablets to dissolve at room temperature; keep medication refrigerated when not in use. Always shake bottles well before using. Distilled water is used to fill the 4 oz. bottles.

CHRONIC COLD SORES / CANKER SORES

Chronic cold sores are usually a direct result of stress. The cause explained in most literature is a virus. Not true! The cause is bacterial. When taking a patch test, the lab technicians may identify viruses and ignore the bacteria which they consider common to everyone–a false assumption.

Copyright 1996 Medisys Research Group, Inc.

Viruses may thrive off the bacteria, but once the bacteria are eliminated, gone are the viruses. The treatment for cold sores is simple and straight forward. In using the medication outlined in the protocol, try to lower your stress levels. Do breathing exercises and try not to worry about everything, especially things you can't do anything about.

What about canker sores in the mouth? Same as cold sores – with the exception of some foods, such as raw pineapple that can cause canker sores.

Not many cankers are attributed to viruses as demonstrated in the development of vaccines that can come from the patient's own canker cells. If bacteria are the host necessary for these viruses to live and grow, hopefully some inquisitive research pioneer will investigate with a daily course of a broad spectrum antibiotic.

Cold Sores and Canker Sore Protocol

Canker sores in the mouth have several causes, but with basically the same symptoms: a mild sore and pain, or a severe sore and severe pain. They can come from biting the lips, from certain foods like fresh pineapple. They can last for a day or two or for a week or longer.

Cold sores on the lips and around the mouth can be short-lived or severe and chronic. Their cause is up for debate, but stress is certainly a factor which affects your immune system ability to fight off the cold sore infection.

Treatment Schedule for Canker Sores

Day 1: Spray the medication into the mouth at the Canker Sore every 15 minutes for the first hour and then once per hour until eight (8) treatments have been made.

Day 2: Spray once per hour until at least six (6) treatments have been made.

*Try not to swallow for a couple of minutes to give the medication time to work. There is no harm when swallowing. The pain will usually subside at least by the end of treatment. However, you should continue to treat for two (2) days regardless. Medication: same as for cold sores (Doxycycline).

Treatment Schedule for Cold Sores

In the first two (2) hours, spray the medication on the affected area and gently rub in with a finger three (3) times (approximately once an hour), after that, spray the medication on the affected area and gently rub in with a finger several times a day. There is no harm in getting medication in the mouth and swallowing.

*Eight (8) of the medicine tablets (Doxycycline) should be put into four (4) oz. liquid containers. Allow three (3) hours for the tablets to dissolve at room temperature; keep medication refrigerated when not in use. Always shake bottles well before using.

Copyright 1996 Medisys Research Group, Inc.

*Continue to treat affected area after it has healed. Healing in most cases will take place within three (3) days unless you are a patient who has experienced chronic cold sores which will require longer treatment. Distilled water is used to fill the 4 oz. bottles.

ECZEMA

Eczema can be found in patients of all ages with some common symptoms such as inflamed rashes, weeping sores, patches of hardened skin, and lots of itching.

If children under twelve years of age appear to have eczema, it may very well be the result of allergies to certain foods, food additives, or something in their home environment. Thus, they need to be tested. There is a product that can be ordered through your local health food store called "child life" which can often control the symptoms of allergies.

For a true eczema condition, follow the treatment protocol and the results can be very rewarding.

Eczema Protocol

Morning: Shower: using liquid non-bacterial soap for washing. Always use a newly washed towel or paper towels to dry with. This is done to avoid recontamination of the skin.

After drying, apply medication topically to all affected areas of the skin. Allow medication to air dry thoroughly before putting on clean clothing worn over affected areas of the skin.

Night: If there have been activities during the day that cause sweating, or getting dirty, another shower is required. If not, in either case, reapplying the medication is required.

Bed sheets and pillow cases should be changed every three (3) days.

IMPORTANT:

- You will not realize a successful treatment if you do not follow the complete protocol.

- For ninety days, no processed sugar in your food, and no natural sugar for the first thirty days. That means no fruit or juices. This is necessary to reduce yeast in the patient's digestive system and help strengthen the immune system.

- At your local health food store, purchase a ninety-day supply of a good probiotic to help in improving your digestive system with good bacteria.

- If the patient is twelve years old or older, purchase a good brand of milk thistle capsules to clean out and rejuvenate the liver. One capsule, taken AM and PM, should be sufficient. For the first two or three weeks the patient may experience some diarrhea and loss of energy. This is a positive response and will subside. Take the milk thistle for a period of six (6) weeks which should be sufficient.

- When the eczema condition has been eradicated, continue the protocol with the topical medication for another two (2) weeks.

Topical Medication:

Four, 100 mg tablets dissolved in a two (2) oz. bottle of distilled water. These tablets are Doxycycline which can be prescribed by your physician. Store the dissolved Doxycycline in the refrigerator when not in use, and always shake the bottle well before applying medication to the skin. Cefdinir may be substituted for Doxycycline.

Note: If your doctor will not prescribe; go to one that will.

NOTE: The absence of sugar in the diet, along with cleansing, will for most patients result in a ten to fifteen-pound loss in weight over ninety days.

UNEXPLAINED SKIN DISEASES

In my twenty-five years of seeing and treating patients, I have seen skin disorders that were frightening to even look at, and had the patient contemplating suicide.

What do you do with these skin disorders? In our case, we threw everything at the problem that we could think of that might have a positive effect.

In other words, we treated them all as though they had psoriasis, plus throwing in an anti-fungal spray for good measure. To this day, I do not know what would cause some of the horrific conditions we have seen, nor do we know why every one of them completely cleared; if it was just part of the therapy, or the entire protocol. We can only say it was almost as much a relief to us as it was for the patient.

Note: Treatment Protocol was the same as for Psoriasis with a sprayed on anti-fungal compound included.

SEBORRHEA

Seborrhea is basically a condition confined to the patient's scalp. In many ways the symptoms imitate those of psoriasis, and are often misdiagnosed as psoriasis.

The treatment protocol for seborrhea is in many ways the same as for psoriasis; except the patient must shave the hair completely from their head. Unless they are willing to do this, there is no chance for success, and that means girls cannot wear a wig, nor can boys wear a hat.

In the protocol there are some subtle differences. Any deviation in the treatment usually translates into no success. I have trained doctors, and once on their own, they have tried to expedite the healing only to discover that they had made things worse or experienced no success with their patients.

This is not to say that more efficient treatments will not be discovered, but there is no substitute for years of research and conventional trials.

Seborrhea Protocol

This is a skin condition, usually associated with the scalp. It is usually identified by severe flaking of the skin along with inflammation and/or a secondary infection. It is often misdiagnosed as Psoriasis which is more difficult to treat. If the treatment protocol we furnish you does not clear the condition, then we will modify the treatment and assume it is Psoriasis and treat it as such. Allow 12 weeks to completely clear and stay clear.

Treatment Schedule

Important: Men and women, unless you are willing to shave your head and keep it shaved until the 12-week treatment schedule is completed, there is nothing we can do to help your condition.

Morning: Wash entire head with clear liquid soap that is NOT anti-bacterial and fragrance free. Rinse head thoroughly and let air dry or use a soft, clean paper towel.

After scalp is dry, spray on medication and gently massage into scalp. Always shake medication bottle before using and store in the refrigerator when not in use.

Mid-day: *Eight (8) medicine tablets (Doxycycline) should be put into four (4) oz. liquid containers. Allow three (3) hours for the tablets to dissolve at room temperature; keep medication refrigerated when not in use. Always shake bottles well before using. The medication to be used can be Doxycycline, 100 mg tabs, or spray on medication powder out of three capsules of Cefdinir, 300 mg; pour small amount at a time on scalp and thoroughly rub into scalp. Distilled water is used to fill the 4 oz. bottles.

Night: Repeat same routine as morning.

Important:

- Change pillowcase three (3) times a week.

- Do not wear a hat until head is healed.

- No processed or natural sugar for ten (10) weeks. Drink no alcohol.

- Take a milk thistle extract capsule twice a day, AM and PM for six (6) weeks.

Copyright 1996 Medisys Research Group, Inc.

- Take a probiotic every day to reduce yeast and help your digestive system.

- Do not expose scalp to the sun as much as possible. You do not want your scalp to sunburn.

- "Vitamin C": 12 years and under – 1,000 mg per day; 13 years and older – 2,000 mg. per day.

- If you must work in the sun, insert a clean paper towel inside hat or helmet to help absorb sweat.

NOTE: The absence of sugar in the diet and cleansing will for most patients result in a ten to fifteen pound weight loss over ninety days.

WOUND HEALING

Wound healing has many bedfellows. There are wound healing centers where successful treatments are used, but still we see patients with diabetes lose their arms and legs from a simple sore or wound. We still see nursing care centers with patients having bed sores and other sores that can spread to other patients.

Why? The answer is simple. The treatment protocols being used take too long to prevent many wound disorders from getting worse and irreversible. Time is not a luxury in favor of many wound conditions.

Thus, the treatment protocols you will find in this book leave the practitioner with no excuse for failure. Our approach to wound healing cannot only eradicate most wounds successfully, but can prevent some conditions from becoming a wound, such as bed sores. Our approach will not eliminate a physician's wound healing practice, but will make it more successful.

Wound Healing Treatment Schedule

Morning: Wash hands with a clear liquid soap that is not antibacterial, and is fragrance free. Then wash affected areas with the same soap. Never use a cloth towel to dry face or other affected areas as you will only re-infect your skin. Paper towels may be used.

Once washed area has air dried, apply medication (Doxycycline) in liquid bottles by spraying on affected areas and rub into the skin thoroughly with fingers and let air dry. Always shake bottle before using.

*Eight (8) of the medicine tablets should be put into four (4) oz. liquid containers. Allow three (3) hours for the tablets to dissolve at room temperature; keep medication refrigerated when not in use. Always shake bottles well before using. Two Cipro tabs, 500 mg each, may be substituted for Doxycycline. Distilled water is used to fill the 4 oz. bottles.

Copyright 1996 Medisys Research Group, Inc.

Day: If area gets sweaty or damp during daytime, use clean paper towels to pat dry.

Night: Shower and repeat morning schedule.

Important:

- Take a good probiotic every day.

- Eat no sugar, processed or natural, or alcohol for ten (10) weeks. This is done to clear the excess yeast from your body.

- Take "Vitamin C": 12 years and under – 1,000 mg per day; 13 years and older – 2,000 mg per day.

- Take a milk thistle extract capsule twice a day, AM and PM, for six (6) weeks.

- Keep clean clothes next to the affected area. VERY IMPORTANT!

- If wound is bleeding or secreting fluid, you may cover with a bandage until wound has formed a solid scab. Once scab has formed, do not cover and continue to spray on medication for five (5) days or longer if wound area still shows inflammation.

- For patients in nursing homes prone to bed sores, massage in medication at FIRST sign of bed sores. Patients in nursing homes who may have infectious sores that may spread to other patients, apply protocol as instructed above.

- The above protocol may be used on diabetic sores to prevent amputation.

SKIN REJUVINATION

From the very beginning of our clinical trials with acne and eczema at the Gresham Medical Center in Oregon, we observed that the faces of acne patients were not only cleared of acne, but their skin was luxurious and beautiful. the skin cells of these patients were rejuvenated! It took approximately ninety days for this rejuvenation to take place. Needless to say, the patients were delighted, and we were amazed.

Today, twenty-five years later, we do not claim to understand why or how this change takes place in the skin cells. How long does this change in the skin cells remain? We don't know, as we have never followed up with those patients. But, because skin cells continue to slough off, we would have to assume that unless the topical medication is continued to be applied, the cell rejuvenation would cease in time.
We did have a sixteen-year-old boy with Cystic acne and extreme scarring, whom we saw eighteen months later, and he was almost totally free of scarring and had vibrant skin.

The protocol for skin rejuvenation is exactly the same as that for acne, and as long as the patient stays on the protocol, the rejuvenation of the skin cells will continue.

NOTE: At some point there may be patients who develop sensitivity to the Doxycycline used topically, and would have to discontinue its use. They can switch to Cefdinir which is

Copyright 1996 Medisys Research Group, Inc.

a third generation of Cefton. Six hundred mg in two ounces of distilled water kept refrigerated should be sufficient if used twice a day AM and PM.

Skin Rejuvenation Protocol

Protocol for skin rejuvenation is the same as for Acne, but with one exception.

<u>Exception</u>: Rejuvenation of the skin cells takes 8-12 weeks as with acne, but in order to maintain the rejuvenation of the skin cells and enjoy the beautiful skin tone, you must continue the protocol.

www.ingramcontent.com/pod-product-compliance
Lightning Source LLC
Chambersburg PA
CBHW081359170526
45166CB00010B/3145